THROUGH THE STORM

by

Aaron G. Perry

authorHOUSE®

AuthorHouse™
1663 Liberty Drive
Bloomington, IN 47403
www.authorhouse.com
Phone: 1-800-839-8640

Published by AuthorHouse 9/17/2012

ISBN: 978-1-4343-3001-7 (sc)
ISBN: 978-1-4678-2432-3 (e)

CONTENTS

Acknowledgement

My parent's love, that's what gave me the strength and courage to face the challenges that have presented themselves to me in this lifetime. The late Mattie Lou Monie and Reverend Albert Perry Senior, you taught me how to push myself far beyond what my eyes could see, and you prepared me to trust even when my doubt stood strong. It is because of your wisdom that I have become the man that I am today, an Ironman.

Preface

The journey to the Ironman will mean many
different things for different people.

For a large percentage of people it will be a goal that will never
materialize because the commitment is far too great.

For some it will mean heartbreak on race day because
the one ingredient missing was how to finish.

For the curious it will be the deciding factor to get up and simply Tri.

And for a very small percentage the Ironman will
be a symbol of great personal achievement.

INTRODUCTION

Through The Storm is a true and inspiring saga of a man who wants more than anything in life to "earn" the title of Ironman Triathlete. At age 42, Milwaukee native Aaron G. Perry, a 15-year insulin dependent diabetic has finally made the commitment to begin training for what would certainly be the most difficult test of physical and mental strength and endurance that he has ever encountered. However, before he can make history, he must first overcome numerous barriers and face many suppressed fears.

Through The Storm shows us all how to triumph when our very foundation is rocked. Told through the lens of his eyes, Perry will inspire everyone to get up and simply (tri).

CHAPTER 1

Why Not Me; Why Not Now?

You can do this Aaron; I know you can, because I believe in you. These words were softly spoken to me by my best friend and soul mate, as I doubted whether or not I would make it through the 2.4-mile swim. With the world's most grueling endurance event scheduled to start in less than 12 hours, I found my confidence fading as quick as the falling night. After a demanding year that involved more than 2,300 hours of high endurance training in preparation for what would certainly be a difficult test of physical and mental strength and endurance, it was down to the final hours before the official start of the Ford Ironman Wisconsin Triathlon, and I was participant #1257.

My Journey began approximately 364 days earlier when I fearfully jumped into the swimming pool to begin the long and tedious process of learning how to swim. I recalled my coach stating, "Aaron, you have so much time it's crazy." He was responding to a question I previously asked, "Do you think I can learn how to swim 2.4 miles in less than a year?" You see, my coach Mark Peterson was one of the best in the Midwest at teaching the art of swimming, and through stroke analysis he helped many athletes learn how to swim at an elite level.

Simply put, he had confidence in me, which I had not found within myself. But, what I did have in my favor was an untapped inner strength combined with my recent discovery that in the 28-year history of the Ironman Triathlon, no African-American diabetic had ever attempted or completed this event.

To put this in better perspective, throughout the past three decades, many African-American diabetic athletes achieved prominence at the collegiate and professional level with honors reaching as high as being inducted into their sports Hall of Fame. But to my surprise, none of these amazing athletes had ever taken on the Ironman competition. As a 17-year insulin-dependent diabetic, I questioned if the sport was too difficult and demanding for diabetics. With more than 2.7 million African-Americans over the age of 20 living with diabetes, these statistics impressed upon me how difficult it would be to accomplish something that no regular Joe or professional athlete has ever attempted.

Emotionally, I had motivated closer to signing up for the Ironman, but deep within my gut, I knew that this challenge would be far greater than anything I had ever attempted in life. I questioned if my untapped inner strength was powerful enough to sustain the tremendous focus and effort required, but then again, for me to become history's first African-American diabetic to complete the world's most difficult ultra endurance event, would not be for fame or fortune, but more of an honor knowing that I accepted a life altering challenge. Suddenly my vision of becoming a pioneer emerged as the defining moment for me to sign up for the Ironman. I had finally found the inspiration to "Just Do It!" I now believed that completing this event would help establish a measurable benchmark that diabetics could use in pushing their fitness to a level beyond comprehension.

Sitting at home with less than 12 hours to go before the biggest event in my 42 years of life, I knew with all my being that I had graduated from a diabetic man trying to lose a little jiggle, to joining the world's elite group of endurance athletes.

I began to reflect upon the all the things I accomplished during the past 364 days, such as the 1,092 before and after meal glucose tests, pushing past the pain of broken ribs, and over 2,300 hours of high endurance training. While walking from my kitchen to the bedroom, I caught a glimpse of myself in the mirror. I smiled at my reflection because during the past 4 years while I sat on my lazy-boy recliner watching the Ironman Triathlon on my 42 inch plasma television, I had marveled at the physiques and the level of conditioning the male and female triathletes were in. And now, with a mere glimpse of myself, I realized I had gotten off my butt and transformed my diabetic body into a chiseled specimen I could be proud of.

As I entered the bedroom, sitting on the edge of the bed was my girlfriend, my love, and my life. She took my hand, placed it near her heart and with that twinkle in her eye stated, "You have come a long way my love, and I'm very proud of what you have become." As the tears welled up in my eyes, the only response I could utter was, "Thank you for your unselfish support throughout this very long and challenging year."

This moment marked the ending of a yearlong battle with numerous physical and psychological challenges that placed a heavy burden on my psyche. Prior to turning in for what would be a long night of tossing and turning in anticipation for what the morning would bring, I said a prayer to God. Only this prayer was different than that of previous nights. Down on bended knees, I asked God to take my diabetes for one day and to simply hold it for me until I crossed the finish line.

CHAPTER 2

Competing With Diabetes

One third of all African-Americans age 20 years or older have diabetes, but don't know it, and millions more have also entered the danger zone called pre-diabetes. Black teens between 10 – 19 years of age are now considered the new face of Diabetes. After years of personally fighting an inner struggle to understand why God gave me this diabetes diagnoses, I now believe his true purpose for my life was revealing itself. But that wasn't always the case!

At age 29, I was the only child out of 6 siblings diagnosed with diabetes. This was a very confusing time for me because I had little knowledge of diabetes. I was a very active, athletic person and had been all my life. I had a strong, fit physique and therefore did not fit the stereotype often associated with diabetics, i.e., being overweight or obese, and living a sedentary lifestyle. This profile simply didn't fit my life.

Prior to being diagnosed with diabetes, I had a throbbing sensation near my kidneys, a persistent cough, frequent urination, and was constantly thirsty. These symptoms lasted for approximately 2 weeks before I sought out answers to what my body was going through.

Realizing that I had to seek medical attention for what I believed to be a bladder infection, I decided to visit an Urgent Care medical facility in the Quad Cities.

I remember walking into the clinic and immediately feeling a sense of relief because I would finally be cured. After meeting with the doctor and answering several questions, he requested that I visit the lab to submit blood work. While sitting and waiting for what seemed to be hours for the results to come back, the nurse finally appeared! She approached me and stated something that I will never forget, "Mr. Perry, you need to walk across the street to the hospital and check yourself into the Emergency Room." I replied, "Why do I need to go to the ER?" The nurse stated, "Your blood work came back and it's registering off our scale of over 450. I'm sorry Mr. Perry, but you are diabetic! Shocked, scared, and feeling hopeless, I began walking the 100 yards to the hospital.

As a former college athlete just 6 years removed from the game, the end of 100 yards would typically mean a score for the team and a roar from the 90 thousand fans that enclosed the stadium. But now, the 100-yard route I ventured on did not include teammates, coaches or fans. I was now all alone and involved in the game of my life.

After checking into the hospital, I remained under physician care for 3 traumatizing days. During this period, I was given diabetes literature to read, and I was taught how to give myself insulin injections. This was very distressing because growing up in the inner city of Milwaukee, Wisconsin, where drug abuse was common; I had vowed never to live a lifestyle that involved drugs and needles. Now, with little say so or control, the very thing I had vowed never to do, would actually be required to save my life.

Over the next 15 years of living with diabetes, my lifestyle involved random glucose testing, and daily insulin injections, a necessity to live. Now age 41, I had made another lifestyle change that included healthier living, and participating in the Ironman Triathlon.

But before I could even consider training my body for a 2.4-mile swim, a 112-mile bike, and a 26.2-mile run, I had to face the reality that

I was not in good health. Over the past 15 years, I had convinced myself that I was doing all that I could to control my diabetes, when in fact my diabetes was controlling me. Prior to beginning my training program, I remember scheduling a physical exam with my personal physician and sharing with him my ambition to do the Ironman. Hoping for words of encouragement, I received a very passive, "Good luck."

Reflecting back at this interaction, I now understood that talking about the Ironman was probably not the best subject to be discussing at that moment. My doctor had just reviewed the results of my lab work which indicated that my blood glucose levels were very high and that I was increasing my risk of diabetes complications such as eye, kidney and nerve damage. Most diabetics know about a simple blood test called hemoglobin A1c that shows where your blood sugar level has been over a 3-month period. The desired A1c goal for diabetics is less than 7% and anything above means a change must be made. My A1c test results were 9.3%, which indicated my diabetes was out of control. I accepted my doctor's passive "good luck" as a wake-up call that I needed to get serious about my health before pursuing the world's most challenging endurance event.

This was my first realization that I was embarking in un-chartered territory. In other words, because 99% of the world's entire population would not even consider attempting the 140.6-mile Ironman Triathlon, why would anyone believe that I would emerge as something special? I lacked discipline, and courage, I had poor control of my diabetes, I was between 25% to 28% body fat, I didn't know how to swim, I had never biked more than 10 miles, had never ran more than 6 miles. And now I was seeking to accomplish something that had never been achieved in our current history.

Suddenly the demand that I was asking of my mind, body and soul would explain why no African-American diabetic had attempted or completed this event. My doctor helped me to understand that training for a long distance triathlon puts healthy people at risk because the challenge is so extreme, and for me having poor control of my diabetes would only increase my risk for health complications.

With 330 days before Ironman, I made a personal commitment to restore personal wellness by moving my diabetes self-care from the backburner to the forefront of my life's busy schedule. I finally met with a nutritionist and a diabetic nurse specialist, and began the process of controlling my diabetes. I truly believe that moving away from random glucose testing, to testing 4-5 times daily, prove to be the single most significant change that altered the course of my diabetes management.

CHAPTER 3

Overcoming Obstacles

With 325 days remaining, I was approximately one month into my swim lessons. Although I faithfully attended each class, the fear of water hovered over my head and became a mental barrier that restricted my forward progress. My swim coach had clearly traveled down this road before because his patience was being tested big time. Although I struggled with getting the technique correct, there were moments in which I sliced through the water like a fish, but was unable to sustain this effort. Recognizing this inconsistency, my coach advised me that he could not help me with the struggles I was exhibiting in the water because they appeared psychological. Other than offering some relaxation exercises, he encouraged me to look within myself for answers.

I appreciated my coach's honest feedback, and I began self-reflecting. I allowed my mind to wander back approximately 37 years. I was 5 years old at the time when my family went to Bradford Beach AKA the lakefront in Milwaukee, Wisconsin. As with previous family outings, I played in the sand before venturing into the waters of Lake Michigan. I was a curious child who often tested limits; at least that's what my parents told me. But on this summer day, I decided to play a game of hide and seek from my family. I walked out into the lake as far as I could and attempted to hide my head under water. As I came up for air, I panicked from drifting out far beyond the shoreline. My small body was no match for the mighty waters of Lake Michigan as the tide had its way with me. I remember looking back at the shore line and believing that everyone was waving at me, when in actuality they were traumatized at the thought of seeing me drown right before their eyes. Although my parents could not swim, I remember seeing their arms slapping the waters as they struggled to move closer to me. Thanks to a courageous bystander, I was rescued and returned to the safe and loving arms of my parents.

Although this near drowning experience occurred almost 4 decades ago, I still remember how tight my mother held me and how much she cried. Not only was this the last time I did anything to make my mother cry, but at age 41, I now realize this was a defining moment in my life and why I avoid living a lifestyle that would make the woman in my life sad. This reflection gave clarity of the man that I have become, and provided me another small fiber of strength.

With 325 days remaining before Ironman, reliving this moment in my past was difficult, but necessary, in order to conquer my fear of water. Letting go was not easy because I felt that I was giving up an intimate memory of my late mother who was killed 2 weeks before my high school graduation. And when you love someone as much as I loved my mother you desperately try and hold onto that memory like a baby clutching a blankie. My mother's memory became my motivation. I began swimming longer and swimming harder, but overcoming my true fear of water would not be realized until I could actually get into the lake and swim, and due to winter fast approaching, that would be 7 long months from now.

It was now October 2004, and not long before the snowy season began. Feeling more confident with other areas of my training, I decided to register for the Green Bay Duathlon, one of Wisconsin's last outdoor cycling and running events before the snowfall.

This event consisted of a 1-mile run, 32-mile bike, and 3.1-mile run. I believed that this would be a good training event and would give my confidence a boost. I convinced 2 of my close friends to enter this event with me. Johnnie Diamante, a UW-Madison Lieutenant and Fred Conley a UW-Madison Police Officer. Although they had absolutely no desire to do the Ironman, they had agreed to support me in the cycling and running. The day leading up to the Green Bay Duathlon, and hours before we hit the road, I made my first and most expensive training related investment. I purchased a Felt Triathlon Bike, and by the time I had added everything I needed (pimped it out), it set me back $3,500.00.

While driving from Madison to Green Bay, I occasionally peeked at my bike that was secured on my vehicle's bike rack while Fred, Johnnie and I spoke about my Ironman training. They both poked fun at me regarding the 2.4-mile swim portion of the Ironman. I had a hell of a time convincing them I was making progress in the pool, but could not escape the infamous stereotype.

"You know black people don't know how to swim, and we hate getting our hair wet."

Although we all found humor in this, there was one thing they had both agreed on, I was beginning to look fit.

Arriving in Green Bay, we went to the registration area set up outside of Lambeau Field, home of the Green Bay Packers. While walking up to register, we were heckled by a Caucasian male who took it upon himself to remind us of our African-American heritage.

"Awe sh##, here comes the fu##in black guys," he yelled.

Not knowing that Fred and Johnnie were police officers, and I being a former police officer, we simultaneously completed a quick Threat Assessment while he continued to heckle us, and we concluded he was just stupid!

After completing registration, we took a quick bike ride through the City of Green Bay. This was my second time actually riding my new bike and while not being an expert in this area, I knew it was a good purchase. This bike was so fast that I gave it a name, Black Thunder!

After the bike ride, we proceeded to check into our hotel. Thanks to race director Gloria West of Midwest Sports Events, the hotel was free of charge. After settling into our room, we turned on the television and began watching a nail-biting football game between the Wisconsin Badgers and the Penn State Nittany Lions. During the 3rd quarter of this exciting game, the hecklers behavior was mentioned. Suddenly the game was no longer a factor and race relations dominated our discussions. Although we each shared our perceptions of this individual, we concluded that he was in his own way being humorous and that he likely meant no harm.

As nighttime fell and morning arrived, there was little discussion between Fred, Johnnie and I. With less than 1.5 hours away from the start of the duathlon, we were all dialed into our competitive mode. In other words, we had our game faces on! Dressed in the latest brand name cycling gear, we left our hotel room and made a brief stop at the continental breakfast kiosk. Fred and Johnnie loaded up on carbohydrates, while my routine required a slight adjustment. Being diabetic, I did not have the luxury of eating and running. I had my own routine, a ritual if you may! I checked my blood sugars, which registered 67, somewhat lower than I would like heading into a race. I loaded up on one peanut butter bagel and a half-cup of orange juice. I decreased my regular dosage of 10-units to 5-units of Humalog Insulin, because the physical exertion during the duathlon would assist in the burning of glucose.

While walking to the transition area, we were met with a chilly 31 degrees, your typical northern Wisconsin fall morning. After setting up my run-to-bike transition, I made eye contact with Fred and Johnnie who were located in separate areas, and I gave them the traditional African-American "head nod" that symbolized good luck. After completing the national anthem, the first leg of the duathlon (1-mile) run had begun.

Approximately 4 minutes into the run, I passed none other than the heckler! He began yelling,

"I knew it, the black guys are going to win."

No comment was required as I blew past him. I arrived back to the transition area in 7 minutes 47 seconds. Pleased with my time, I began the run to bike transition. As I looked up, I could see Johnnie already exiting the bike transition and into the 31-mile bike. Fred arrived shortly after and we both were out of the transition area seconds apart. Immediately into the bike ride I regretted not having cycling gloves. The chilly air was already taking a toll on my fingers, but I was focused and into my groove. As I approached mile 3, I was already feeling heavy legs. For an insightful moment, I pondered how far I was from being in shape for the112-mile Ironman bike that was now approximately 325 days away, but I kept pushing on!

As I approached mile 5, I began descending down a rather steep hill. Suddenly, an unexpected sharp corner appeared and I realized I was moving far too fast to navigate the turn. I immediately applied slight pressure onto my brake, which sent my rear wheel into a skid. As I attempted to correct the skid, I completely lost control of my bike and proceeded to slam into the ground.

I attempted to shift my body out of the path of other cyclist who were also descending down the hill, but the severe back pain prevented me from moving. Unable to breath, I felt that I most likely sustained a serious injury, but soon after a sense of safety was felt after a DePere Wisconsin Police Officer appeared. It seemed only seconds ago that I had passed him as he was directing traffic, and now he had his hand slightly grazing my chest while shielding me with his body as he waved other cyclists away from my direction. I heard him call out from his shoulder radio to his dispatcher to send a paramedic. By now, I believed I had suffered a broken back and a collapsed lung. Still unable to catch my breath I could not answer any of the questions the officer asked.

"Are you all right? Can you move? Where are you injured?"

The only response I could render was a nod of my head while barely whispering,

"I can't catch my breath."

The officer told me to relax and informed me that the paramedics were en route. I caught a glimpse of my brand new bike and it appeared intact. The officer must have observed my painful arch of the head as I checked out my bike. He stated, "Don't worry about your bike, I will secure it at the police department."

Now I knew what it felt like to be on the other side of the fence. As a former police officer, I had responded to numerous accidents. I recalled approaching victims to render aid, assessing the extent of their injury and, most importantly, assuring them that they would be safe.

Hmm!! Now I understood what my parents meant. As a youngster, they would often state,

"Son, be good to people and it will come back to you."

It seemed as though the paramedics arrived right away. They performed all of the necessary safety procedures that I myself had learned during the EMT training I received in the Police Academy. They secured my head, strapped me down, and I was off to the hospital. All in all, I gave the Officer and the Paramedics a well-deserved A+.

During the short drive to the hospital, I remember feeling a sense of sadness because I believed my injuries were not only severe, but they would interfere with my swimming lessons. Strapped in the ambulance with severe chest and back pain, I decided that no matter what the extent of my injuries were, it would not stop my journey to becoming an Ironman. Reflecting back on this moment, I realized why so few people become an Ironman. It demands more than what most people are willing to give!

Upon arriving at the hospital, I was met by several nurses who assisted with transferring me to a medical bed and began assessing my injuries. My flow of breathing was still difficult, but during the assessment I was able to advise the medical personnel where the pain was located. The pain I previously felt in my back had shifted to my chest area. Although I was in serious pain, I was relieved to have some use of my back. Not broken was my diagnosis! But I needed to hear it from the doctor. I found the ER nurses to be extremely patient and comforting, but after a brief exam, I was taken to the x-ray room where I was not as fortunate with the X-Ray Tech. The young and very attractive female advised me to perform certain movements that I simply could not perform. She directed me to sit up straight, but the pain would not allow me to move. I advised her that my pain level was around 9. As a trained medical professional, she should have known that 10 meant serious pain, but she either didn't know, or she simply didn't care!

She proceeded to inform me that she could not complete her task if I didn't respond. I remember stating, "I'm trying, but I'm in severe pain and can't move." She proceeded to state, "With all those muscles you should be able to move."

Now, back in my college days I would have assumed she was flirting with me, but as an older, wiser adult who thinks above his waistline, I knew she was not complimenting me by any stretch of the imagination.

My second attempt to "sit up straight" brought on more pain in my chest area and from the look on my face she must have finally realized I could not move. When she requested assistance from another nurse, her tone of voice was less than professional. I soon realized she was just as impatient with her own co-workers, and for a moment I thought maybe she was related to the Heckler. After finally completing the x-rays, I found myself still in severe pain but was happy to leave the company of the very attractive X-Ray Tech from hell. Boy, what a waste!

While waiting for my x-ray results, I began to compare how long I had been at the hospital to how long it would have taken Fred and Johnnie to complete their first duathlon. I estimated for a 1-mile run, 30-mile bike and 3.1-mile run the average time of completion would likely be 2 hours 10 minutes.

With the exception of a few newbie's such as Fred and Johnnie, this time of year (the fall) is a time most athletes have just completed their summer season of competing in marathons and triathlons and therefore their conditioning level is still pretty solid. It was a safe bet that Fred and Johnnie had crossed the finish line and by now were wondering what was taking me so long!

The ER nurse assisted me by calling their cell phone to inform them of my whereabouts. She advised me that my friends had already been informed of my accident by other race participants, but didn't know where I had been transported. The nurse provided them with an update on my condition and they were given directions to the hospital.

The doctor arrived shortly after and discussed the results of my x-rays. I braced myself in anticipation for his diagnosis. He stated, "Mr. Perry, you have a fracture of the 4th and 5th rib." He provided me with a prescription for pain and gave me some self-care instructions. "Thanks Doc!" I replied, as I shook his hand. Relieved that I had no other injuries, I gathered what was left of my cycling outfit (after being cut off my body) and I walked to the waiting room. As I sat waiting for Fred and Johnnie to arrive, to my surprise I observed a couple (age groupers) I recognized from the duathlon. They were preparing to exit the ER with the boyfriend pushing the girlfriend in a wheelchair. Her leg had a brace on it that reflected a knee injury. I wondered at what point of the race she had suffered her injury. As the very fit couple passed by me, we made eye contact. No words were necessary, just eye contact and silence reflected our frustration.

Johnnie and Fred arrived and were quickly debriefed on what had happened. Out of respect for me being injured, I found Johnnie to be more cautious and reserved with bragging about completing his first duathlon. Fred on the other hand, didn't give a crap! He talked so much stuff that you would have thought he had won the darn race. After trying to convince them for several years to participate in an event with me, I was proud of them both for finishing.

During the drive back to Madison, I realized what amazing friends I have. In between coping with fractured ribs that hurt like heck, and Fred's trash talking, it was mentioned that my quest to become an Ironman had helped turn a once impossible barrier into an inspiring accomplishment. In recognizing the set back I suffered, both Johnnie and Fred encouraged me to move past this barrier, and attack this injury as simply another opportunity to amaze myself.

CHAPTER 4

Putting Life In Perspective

My journey towards becoming an Ironman would definitely continue, but living with diabetes and recovering from fractured ribs would make it more difficult. With the 2.4-mile swim less than 325 days away, I knew the challenge of learning how to swim had become more complicated. After researching fractured ribs online, I learned that it could take a minimum of 6 months to heal completely. That's 6 months for a healthy person! When you're diabetic, your immune system is compromised which slows the healing process down. Therefore, I had anticipated that it could take between 7 to 8 months for my ribs to completely heal. Although I wanted more than anything to earn the title of Ironman, I accepted that improving my health would be the most important decision at that time.

From mid October 2004 through January 2005, my training had come to a complete halt. During this period, I must admit, I attempted to test my injury in hopes that a miracle healing had occurred, but with each attempt to swim, bike or run came a painful reminder that rib injuries needed time to heal. As I reluctantly learned the art of being patient during this time, I also realized that training under unpleasant emotional and mental circumstances only created negative motivation.

What had consumed my every thought and dominated most of my conversations, the Ironman Triathlon was finally put into perspective. I reconnected with family and friends over the Thanksgiving, Christmas and New Year's holidays and was reminded of what's really important. As I found a peaceful place within my life, I became more patient and accepting of my circumstance. Although I was no longer talking about triathlons, I couldn't escape the question, "How is your training going?" With all the positive energy flowing in my direction, I had hoped that this would somehow speed up my recovery. There were several close friends who were living their desire to be a triathlete through me and had placed me on a pedestal that I had not yet earned! Talk about pressure to heal and resume my training! I definitely felt it.

Sadly during this period, my younger brother made a serious error in judgment that ultimately cost him his freedom. He was arrested in Rhinelander, Wisconsin, and charged with possession of a controlled substance with intent to deliver. As a former police officer, I knew all too well how organized drug dealers operate. My brother was not an organized drug dealer; instead he was a bright person with a promising future who tried to make a quick buck. As a character witness, I testified at my brother's sentencing hearing. I stated to the judge that I understood the seriousness of the crime committed, but I also took the time to help the court understand my family's dynamics.

I shared with the judge how my late mother instilled positive values and a strong sense of family and community in the older siblings, but my younger brother who was only 6 years old when my mother passed away, did not have a maternal figure guiding him through his young adult years. I informed the judge that being an older brother, I failed to pass on to my brother the lessons I received during my upbringing and instead he was left to fend for himself. I assured the judge that whatever the outcome of the court's decision, I would step up to the plate and become more of a role model in my brother's life.

Prior to handing down the sentence, the judge advised my brother that he would have received a 12-year sentence, but believing that having a positive family member involved in his life would help in the long run. My brother was given a 4-year prison sentence, and with his time already served would lessen this to 2 years in prison for good behavior.

As the New Year rolled in, I was finally able to resume my training program with a different perspective on family and life. Because I was unable to train for approximately 70 days, I had lost strength, endurance and most important I had lost confidence. But this time around would be different because during my recovery period I had developed a better relationship with God, a relationship I under-appreciated prior to getting injured. I now believed that with God all things were possible.

CHAPTER 5

How I Got My Groove Back

It was now January 6, 2005, and 248 days before The Ironman Wisconsin Triathlon, and my back was up against the wall. I eagerly resumed my swimming lessons with my coach Mark, but I could sense that something was different with him. He didn't seem as confident in his ability to teach me how to swim 2.4 miles. Maybe he was concerned with the fact that my fractured ribs had not been given sufficient time to heal, but I needed to get back into the water. I began swimming with him 2 times per week and during each drill he pushed me extremely hard, as a coach should. From January through April, my swimming had improved, but keeping it real with myself, I was still a long way from swimming 2.4 miles, thus not earning the right to move onto the 112-mile bike, the 2nd stage of the Ironman Triathlon. To put this in better perspective, 87 laps in the pool that I trained in equaled 2.4 miles. I was only able to swim 20 laps before my arms and leg muscles reached physical failure. Needless to say, I was a long way from my goal. I began praying a great deal because I knew I needed the assistance of a higher power.

April 7, 2005, came around and I was 178 days away from Ironman. With my swimming improving ever so slightly, I made the decision to hire a triathlon coach to help increase my core strength and improve my cycling and running stamina. I contacted the University of Wisconsin Sports Medicine Program and began my relationship with Jude Sullivan. Immediately I liked Jude's presence because his mannerisms were very similar to mine, soft-spoken and easily approachable. These same qualities were once present within Mark, my swim coach, but had faded from lesson to lesson.

With the help of Jude, I immediately began to have a clear sense of direction with my training. Jude helped me understand what I had gotten myself into in terms of my pursuit to become an Ironman. There were so many aspects of my training that I was not made aware of until our relationship began. Jude designed 3 separate training programs for me that consisted of 9 weeks each. He was the first person to suggest that I participate in a half marathon, 2 sprint triathlons and a half Ironman prior to participating in the full Ironman Triathlon. Although I trusted Jude, I truly did not believe I could achieve this level of fitness. But again, I trusted him even more than I trusted my own abilities. Jude helped me believe that by participating in these smaller events one at a time I would begin building confidence and improve on areas needing improvement.

With 189 days of training down and 5 months remaining before Ironman, I had begun to wonder what obstacles remained for me. Armed with a more clear sense of direction and purpose, I shifted my training regimen into another gear, a strange place for me because I had never pushed myself to this point. Whether training indoors or out, I was in full throttle, and the physical changes were becoming apparent.

My health had improved and my hemoglobin A1C was now below 7.0, which was a major victory for me because I was finally in control of my diabetes. A far cry from the 9.3 range I was at 189 days ago.

Other noticeable changes were my skin complexion had seen dramatic improvements a direct result of the high amounts of H20 I had consumed during my training. I was sleeping better during the night, and my abdominal area went from resembling a case to resembling a six-pack.

Yeah Baby!

With all the physical changes occurring in my life, the one area of improvement I was most proud of was how my spirit had begun to positively influence my family and friends. Everyone was discussing scheduling doctor appointments and beginning to exercise on a regular basis. The inspiration I had on my loved ones was so surreal that I began thinking outside the box.

"Wow! Could I have this kind of an impact on ordinary folks living with diabetes?"

"How many of the millions of people struggling to control their diabetes could I inspire by simply crossing the finish line in the world's most grueling endurance event?"

I had already achieved a personal victory by gaining better control of my diabetes, and I hoped that my ability to move my diabetes care from a dangerous place would serve as an example that empowers other (Type 1) or (Type 2) diabetics.

With 5 months remaining before the Ironman, I realized that I had previously been looking at the glass as half empty when in fact it was half full. God was answering my prayers by guiding me towards people, places and situations that I had yet to realize. I was given a more positive attitude with a powerful force of determination that would get me through the tough times that awaited me.

CHAPTER 6

Pushing On In Spite Of...

As March rolled in, Johnnie, Fred and I hooked up again and had begun putting in some serious miles on our chosen running shoes in preparation for a popular running event called the Syttende Mai. This is a 20-mile very hilly run that starts in downtown Madison, Wisconsin, and ends in downtown Stoughton, Wisconsin. Within weeks, we were pushing out 8 to 10-mile runs 3 times weekly and a 15 to 20 mile run once weekly.

As the month of April rushed in, it seemed to leave just as quickly. It seemed like only yesterday that Fred, Johnnie and I had begun increasing our mileage. With Syttende Mai being one week away, my thoughts were, if I could finish in a good time, I'd establish a good running base and have a better indication of my cardiovascular fitness level.

I began my weeklong preparation that included a pasta supper each night (carb loading) and consuming of lots of H2O. My other preparation required me to cut back on my insulin regimen dosage.

Instead of 3 injections daily, I cut down to 2 per day, but increased the number of times I checked my blood glucose levels from 4 to 8.

May 2, 2004, and it's race day! I arrived at approximately 6:00 am to register and to give myself and my nerves time to settle down. I located Fred and Johnnie around 6:30 am, in the midst of approximately 1,000 participants. With the temperature around 70 degrees and a light breeze blowing, the brothers were together again just like the Green Bay Duathlon. After taking turns stretching one another, I did a quick check of my blood sugars that read 110, which was normal range. We gave each other high fives and wished one another good luck. Following the national anthem, the race was on. After navigating through the pack of runners and completing mile 2, I checked my heart rate and determined I was running around a 7-minute pace, far too fast to maintain! I reminded myself that this was a 20-mile run, and I needed to run a smart race. I had previously estimated that it would take me 3 hours to complete the race, providing everything went as planned, but now that I was in it, time did not matter, only finishing mattered.

As I got through the first 10 miles, my legs felt good, but my thoughts could not escape the comparison to what these 10 miles would feel like following a 2.4-mile swim and a 112-mile bike. I quickly abandoned all thoughts of the Ironman Triathlon and shifted my focus back in the moment. It seemed from mile 10 to 15, this race route covered every major hill there was. My heart monitor was holding steady at 160, and with approximately 5 miles remaining, my time was 2 hours 40 minutes to be exact. Johnnie was out of sight from the time the race began, and I could see Fred approximately 150 yards ahead of me. No need to try and catch him because for one, I didn't think I had it in me and for two, I was simply trying to hold my pace and finish.

As I passed mile 17, I began to feel my diabetic body searching for energy from any cell it could find. With 3 miles remaining, I could feel my body giving all that it had. With every step and with every pound of the pavement I kept telling myself, "Aaron, keep moving forward." As I passed mile 19, I knew I would finish, but it became the longest mile I had ever run. As I passed through the downtown area, there were many spectators yelling encouragements. But just like most small towns that

I had ever visited, there was always one bigot present. With 300 yards remaining and barely holding on to the finish, I heard this loud smoker's voice yell,

"Hey black boys, you still have 30 miles to go."

It seemed as if the loud music had stopped and the cheering came to a halt as I passed by. Now, I don't know what happened to this individual, but I believe the spectators that were proud of their community chewed him a new butt. Thank you Stoughton residents!

My time of completion was 3 hours 34 minutes and my heart rate average was 157. I checked my post-race glucose levels and my meter read a very low 47, which explained the light-headedness! After locating the refreshments stand and eating several orange slices, I allowed myself to finally celebrate because I had cleared one major hurdle towards building the endurance necessary to become an Ironman. As I met up with Johnnie and Fred, they both had impressive times of 2 hours 35 minutes and 3 hours 25 minutes respectively. Because of our successful completion, we immediately discussed participating in the Madison Marathon that was less than 3 weeks away.

As the sweet smell of spring filled the air, it was time to move my indoor cycling to the great outdoors. After hearing about the challenging 112-mile Ironman bike route that included 6,900 feet of climbing, I would finally get a chance to experience it up close and personal. This would also be the first opportunity to ride my bike outdoors since my accident in the Green Bay Duathlon.

Fred and I had participated in spinning classes offered at our local fitness center from mid January to the present, and with a slight cycling base established, we were ready to hit the road. The weekends were designated as our long cycling days because we didn't have to navigate heavy traffic. Our first planned bike ride, we stayed true to our game plan of hitting the pavement by 6:00 am. We rode from Madison to Verona and back to Madison, a 32-mile ride that took about 2 hours. This was my first time riding a bike this distance and although it was fun, my initial impression was. "Darn it! This is going to be rough."

I was thrilled with completing 32-miles the first time out, but my reality was that in the Ironman I would still have 80 miles to go with the toughest terrain ahead of me. Thirty two miles in 2 hours was unacceptable! The time became a major factor, and I believed I had begun stressing over it. Ironman rules stipulate that participants have until 5:30 p.m. to complete the 112-mile bike course. Just when I thought my biggest challenge would be swimming 2.4-miles in less than 2 hours 20 minutes, I now had something new to fret about.

Determined to become more confident and competitive, I took full advantage of my muscular legs and my improved cardiovascular health. I made significant strides and ultimately developed the endurance that enabled me to extend my training rides from 32-miles to 72-miles. The Ironman bike course consisted of riding from Madison to Verona, (16 miles) completing two 40 miles loops that ventured into the smaller more rural communities of Verona, Mt. Vernon, Mt. Horeb, Cross Plains and back to Verona, (80 miles), and then back to Madison for a total of 112 miles.

By now I was left to bike on my own because my new training program required 60 to 70-mile bike rides followed by an 8 to 15 mile run. Fred had politely abandoned me during the weekend rides because he had no desire or reason to push himself this distance. I had clearly become a much stronger cyclist over the previous 2 months and I began linking up with athletes from different triathlon clubs because they were the pros, and if you want to be the best that you can be, you must train with the best.

Each time I had the opportunity to ride with different clubs, I was able to knock off about 10 – 20 minutes on my time. Although I had yet to ride the entire 112-mile course, I had begun to believe that I could do it. With my cycling time improving, my anaerobic heart rate stabilizing within the designated zone and my blood sugars responding favorably to the high endurance training, my confidence was growing, and I was in hot pursuit of my courage. I knew that if I could control the things I had the power to control, I would put myself in a position to succeed at the bike stage of the Ironman Triathlon.

CHAPTER 7

The Power To Withstand

With approximately 96 days remaining before Ironman, things had begun to change. People had begun to change. During previous bike rides through the rural communities of Mt. Horeb and Cross Plaines, I had encountered some hostility from some of the small town folks, but had believed it was due to the fact that some motorists hated sharing the rode with a cyclist. Some would often express their strong dislike by placing thumb tacks around portions of the Ironman route causing numerous flat tires. But on this particular weekend day, I remember singing the tunes of a Mariah Carey's song while approaching the village of Mt. Horeb. As I hummed the lyrics, "Don't let the world break me tonight,"

Bam! Right in the back of the head.

As this object hit me, I swerved off the road. At this time I saw 3 punks driving a piece of crap car not fit for the road and yelling many obscenities. After gathering myself together, I began to wipe off the substance that had been hurled at me. It was at this time I realized I had been hit in the back of the head by a cup/can of beer.

Although I was disturbed by their actions, I still had another 40 plus miles to go. As I traveled the remaining distance, my "Threat Assessment" was very high. Every car that approached from the rear made me cringe. In my many years on this earth that I've encountered hatred and racism, this was by far the first time I truly felt vulnerable and completely butt-naked. As I arrived at the Mt. Horeb stop-n-go station where many cyclists stop to use the bathroom and replenish fluids, I was able to link up with other cyclists for the remainder of my bike ride.

Drenched with the smell of alcohol, I felt compelled to explain to my fellow riders why the odors of intoxicants were emanating from my person. After all, I didn't want them thinking that I was cycling under the influence. I simply offered that someone must have tossed a cup of beer out the window, and I was the un-intended victim. But being a good Christian person, I decided to keep my real thoughts to myself.

I managed to keep my composure as I had done many times with prior incidents. What I had appreciated during the remainder of my ride was hearing other cyclists talk about their goals and challenges. It became apparent that as I interacted with people who shared similar goals and interests, race or gender didn't matter.

Upon completing my 70-mile bike ride, I decided to postpone my usual 8 to 10-mile run and complete it the following day. I instead contacted my friend Ken Snoddy, a City of Madison Police Officer and African-American male. I needed to debrief about this frightening incident and was hoping for a different perspective.

Early into the conversation, I realize it was difficult discussing this issue with Ken without bringing in a history of bigoted behaviors we both experienced during our early adulthood. After seeking a different perspective from some old college buddies, they also challenged my desire to continue cycling on that very road in which a mere 5 inches separated me from vehicles driven by a few hate yielding people.

Clearly all the advice received from my close friends was well intended, but at the end of the day, I chose to fall back on the lesson my parents had instilled in me when they would state, "Son, even when your actions are justified, they must always be dignified." As with other unfortunate dilemmas I found myself in, I had once again taken their advice and found a different perspective on this incident. I concluded that although I was dazed by this unfortunate experience, this one incident could not alter the course of my Ironman journey.

And so the Christian man that I am took the high road and pressed forward!

CHAPTER 8

Conquering Suppressed Fears

It was now mid May and the local lakes had warmed to approximately 68 degrees. The time had finally arrived for me to face head on my fear of water. My swim coach offered a lake swim class for Ironman hopefuls and I was among the first to register. The class met from May 25, 2006, through September 2, 2006, ending approximately 9 days before Ironman. The high cost of the class, $250.00 was a small price to pay for the confidence I was hoping to gain, especially considering I made the decision to participate in the Quad Cities Triathlon that was scheduled for June 18, 2006, and less than 3 weeks away.

A 600-yard swim was all that was required for the swim portion of the Quad Cities Triathlon, and I simply was not confident I could do it. During the winter months, I did my swim training at a number of fitness center pools in which the water was 5-6 feet deep. On most days, if I felt fatigue, I would simply stand in the water or rest on the wall. But swimming in a 75-foot deep lake meant no walls to grab onto, and water too deep to stand in. Simply put, I needed to be able to swim this distance, and I had 28 days to figure out how.

As the lake swim classes began, I clearly sucked! No confidence, no pride, no nothing. My swim coach began challenging me to go further with each class. He would give the class a simple task to swim out to the buoy and back. The buoys were positioned about 100 feet from the shoreline, and with each instruction, I would swim out with the class. However, approximately 50 feet out, I would turn around and swim back to shoreline while the rest of the class completed the task. I had no confidence, and the fear I internalized had consumed me. I remember my coach stating, "Aaron, I want you to look out as far as you can see and know that your courage is on the other side of the lake. Within one month, I expect you to be swimming to the other side of the lake and back twice. This challenge issued by my coach would equal the distance of a 1.2-mile swim.

With each class thereafter, I began swimming further from the shoreline and with more confidence. This was a major accomplishment for me, but I had fallen far behind other swimmers, which meant I was disappointing my coach. One of the qualities I admired in Mark was his strong sense of safety for his swimmers, but having me fall so far behind other swimmers during the first three weeks of lake swim classes meant my coach was put in a position to either watch me and ignore the group or vice versa. I knew deep inside I was becoming a liability, but what I had not realized was that my coach had reached the end with me. Even though he had begun to lose confidence in me, I gained confidence and had begun to believe that that I could complete the 600-yard swim. With three days remaining before my first ever triathlon, taking ownership of this level of confidence was significant for me.

I guess in life, someone's loss (confidence) is your gain!

The day before the Quad Cities Triathlon had finally arrived, and with my best friend and soul mate sitting next to me, we were on the interstate I-39 en-route to Davenport, Iowa. This was my first road trip as a triathlete wannabe, and I was scared as hell! Although I tried to mask my nerves by singing my favorite Usher and Mariah Carey tunes, my girlfriend simply stroked my shoulders with her soft hands, which provided the reassurance I needed. I thanked God for sending this woman to me!

As we passed through Illinois and entered the state of Iowa, it was sort of a home coming for me because I had spent much of my 20's learning life's lessons while attending college in Iowa. Driving up to the Holiday Inn, the official sight of the Quad Cities Triathlon registration brought back many memories. This is where I worked during the summer of both my junior and senior years of college. My official title at the Holiday Inn was Linen Person, but there was one worker in particular who insisted on referring to me as, "The Linen Boy." The worker that I'm referencing was an openly gay female whom stood 6'4" and weighed a biscuit from 300 lbs. She never knew this, because I never stated it to her face, but I also had established a name for her,

"Big Dude".

From my first day on the job, she had it in for me. I later found out through other workers that "Big Dude" felt threatened by me because several of the females were attracted to the new guy. I got the message loud and clear while working one day when "Big Dude" apparently witnessed me having a conversation with one of the female staff. She sent the following message through a co-worker, "Tell the Linen Boy! That these are all my girls and that's all I have to say." Needless to say, I decided to keep my social life out of the workplace. Hmm…memories, memories….

Walking into the front lobby to register for the triathlon I noticed the place looked exactly as it did 10 years earlier. After completing registration, we checked into our room, unpacked our bags and we were off for a tour of Davenport, Iowa. After years of sharing different stories with my girlfriend about my college days, I was finally able to share it up close and personal, and it seemed very intimate to share this with my best friend. We toured my old dorm room, the gymnasium and the classrooms. She took the trip down memory lane, and she even allowed me to brag about the athlete I used to be. After reminiscing, it was time to get down to the real business at hand. I drove out to West Lake Park, the actual sight where the triathlon took place. I needed to see the transition area, but more importantly, I had to see the actual swim course.

Staring from the shoreline, the 600-yard swim course looked very intimidating, and seeing it up close gave my body a chill that I cannot explain. Even though the race was still 13 hours away, I felt like I had already earned the title Triathlete. I believe I felt this way because after years of talking about doing a triathlon, I had finally arrived.

After grabbing supper, we headed back to the hotel for the evening. The alarm went off at 5:00 am, and after showering and getting all my gear packed, we were off to the park. We were among the first to arrive before a steady stream of vehicles started pouring into the parking lot. As the sun came up, the park came alive. The music played loud and the triathletes started going through their rituals. Although this was not the Ironman, it had the same electricity, only on a smaller scale. After placing my bike in the transition area, I proceeded to the body-marking tent to get branded. Number 936 on the arm and number 41 (age) on my left leg. With less than 30 minutes before the first wave of swimmers hit the water, I squeezed into my wetsuit. Still about 12 pounds heavier than I had planned to be for Ironman, but the wetsuit disguised it pretty good. My final preparation was completed, I said a prayer, kissed my girlfriend, and I was off to the swim course.

After a brief announcement from Eric Sarno, the race director, the first wave had begun. I was in wave number 5 and before long my wave was released. I was obviously nervous as I entered the water and I proceeded to walk out as far as I could before I was finally into my stroke. The water was initially chilly on my face but became unnoticeable as my adrenalin kicked in. Just 5 minutes into my first triathlon swim, I had found a rhythm, just like my coach stated I would. I pressed forward and I tried to remember everything my coach had taught me. As I came around the third of 6 buoys, I began to feel slightly fatigue, but I had my sights fixed on the shoreline and with each stroke I came closer and closer to completing the swim. As I approached the shore, I could hear the crowd screaming, and within seconds I was out of the water, (16 minutes) "I did it! I did it! I whispered silently to myself.

Jogging towards the bike transition, I saw this big smile on my girlfriend's face. As I passed by I heard her yelling,

"Yea, you did it".

I smiled at her, pumped my fist and pushed on. I quickly got out of the wetsuit and transitioned into my cycling gear. As I mounted my bike, I remember feeling very confident. Approximately 3 miles into the bike, I had begun to pay attention to the participants already completing the 15-mile bike ride. They represented all shapes, sizes and genders. Some extremely fit and others just simply tri-ing. As I approached the 10-mile point, I began to drive my legs into the pedals just like in spinning class. My legs felt solid, but a long way from a 112-mile bike. As I approached the finish line, I caught a glimpse of the clock, (55 minutes), and I was very pleased with this time.

After dismounting my bike, I quickly checked my glucose levels, which registered a safe 105. I proceeded to change into my running shoes and was off into the 3.1-mile run. My legs felt heavy during the first 2 minutes, but then my training kicked in. Running is my strength, and it soon showed. As I approached the only hill on the route, I pumped my arms hard and in rhythm with each step I took. The run seemed effortless as I approached the finish line in a full stride.

Wow!

I had just completed my first triathlon in 1 hour 34 minutes, and I felt great! When I found my girlfriend, she was just as happy and proud as I was. Pumped up and full of confidence, I had mentally committed to registering for the Aurora High Cliff Half Ironman Triathlon the following weekend.

As I gathered my personal belongings and prepared to depart Iowa, it really hit home as to why people do triathlons. For me personally, there was no prize money and no trophy, just the personal satisfaction of being called a triathlete, and it felt awesome!

My next challenge was approximately one week away and I couldn't wait. Consisting of a 1.2-mile swim, 56-mile bike, and 13.1-mile run, the half Ironman would be a tough event. I couldn't wait to return home so I could log onto the computer and officially sign up. Deep down inside, I knew I needed to sign up before my newly found confidence faded.

The ride back to Madison was completely different than my ride to Davenport. No masking of fear. Instead, I was heading home with a new found confidence. I obviously had the physical ability to complete a triathlon, but it wasn't until I actually tried, that I realized that ability was in me. I now understood what Stella felt when she got her groove back. For me, I had found my triathlon swagger and I was full of confidence.

I would have never known this feeling had I not made the attempt.

With one week of time separating me from the Aurora High Cliff Half Ironman, I knew I had to make the most of each day. Having my first test of swimming in a triathlon go exceptionally well, I had to remind myself to keep things in perspective, because there was a big difference between swimming 600 yards and 1.2 miles. Although the Quad Cities Triathlon swim brought out an ability that I already had within me, I also knew the Half Ironman swim of 1.2-miles would be a test of my true swimming ability. Completing this event would move me physically and mentally one more step closer to achieving the full Ironman swim of 2.4-miles.

With approximately 75 days remaining before Ironman Wisconsin, things were shaping up very well. I had resumed my lake swim classes following the Quad Cities Triathlon, and there was a noticeable difference in my confidence level. For the first time since beginning swim lessons, I completed every drill my coach had given. Although my speed still lagged far behind the majority of the class, I stuck with each drill and I eventually caught up with everyone. No stopping early, no turning around, and no cutting drills short.

With 5 days down and less than 48 hours remaining before the Aurora High Cliff Half Ironman, I decided that a 2-day taper would be wise. During the previous 5 days of training, I completed a total of 6 miles of lake swimming, 120 miles on the bike and 20 miles of running. Nutrition wise, I had managed to take in a pasta supper each evening. With my diabetes insulin regimen, I scaled back to 2 insulin injections daily as opposed to 3. Completing my first triathlon had clearly put my training on another level.

In the blink of an eye and with great anticipation, I was on the road for the second time in a week heading out of town for another triathlon. The destination was the beautiful Shorewood Wisconsin Park, located in northwestern Wisconsin approximately 15 miles from Appleton.

During the 2-hour drive to Shorewood, my girlfriend and I talked about how much fun we were having on my journey to the Ironman. With minimal distractions to date, I was happy I had chosen to train for the Ironman Wisconsin Triathlon. As we arrived in Shorewood Wisconsin, the triathlon fever was definitely in the air as many triathletes descended on the park to register. Upon completing registration, I ventured down to the swim course to see what I was up against. This was definitely further, and much more of an intimidating swim course than Quad Cities was... at least that's what I had concluded.

I sat near the shoreline and envisioned myself swimming the 1.2-mile course. My girlfriend respected my moment with nature by choosing to stay in the vehicle. She seemed to always know what I needed and when I needed it. To be honest, I found the swim course to be very frightening, but having my rock nearby providing emotional support helped to keep my confidence high.

After scouting out the course, we headed to Applebee's Restaurant for supper. I had managed to sneak in one last pasta dinner, hoping to store that extra glycogen in my tank. I figured that the Half Ironman would take around 6 hours to complete, and anything I could store in reserves would certainly be needed.

Upon finishing supper, we returned to the hotel room for the evening for a solid night of sleep. At approximately 1:00 am, I realized that staying in a cheap hotel on a Saturday night was not a good idea. (Note to self, spend the money next time.) It seemed every party person had, like me, found a cheap place to stay for the night.

There was loud music thumping from car stereos, and intoxicated people walking the hallways totally insensitive to the idea of respecting other's privacy.

I must say that when I left the hotel at 5:30 am, I had entertained the devious thought of pulling the hotel's fire alarm just to upset people, but it was just a thought!

Arriving at the park, I began my ritual of setting up my transition area. Preparing next to me was #377. I don't remember his name, but I will always remember his passion for competition. This man (age grouper) had fractured his elbow 6 days prior, but was still determined to participate. For a moment, I struggled to understand swimming and cycling with a fractured elbow, but then again many people struggle to understand why a diabetic would do a triathlon. Assisting a fellow triathlete put on his wetsuit and strap on his bike helmet helped me to further understand my passion and determination to becoming an Ironman.

After assisting my new friend, I put on my wetsuit, checked my glucose levels which read 140, and I headed down to the water. I was placed in wave 7, and before I knew it, my wave was up next. I recall catching a glimpse of my girlfriend seconds before my wave was released, and I gave her the thumbs up! As the horn sounded, I entered the water to begin the 1.2-mile swim. I immediately began taking wide strokes to relieve some of the crowding, a tip that I learned from my mentor, Dino Lucas, a 5-time Ironman Triathlete.

Although I accidentally elbowed many people while stroking wide, I knew it was part of the competition and nothing personal. As I approached the opening of the marina, I immediately realized how the rocks surrounding the marina had blocked the view of the lake. Staring at the lake from shore was intimidating, but rounding the marina wall and being exposed to the entire lake made me buckle down for what I thought would be a long swim.

"A very massive, yet beautiful lake. Here I come."

As I passed the first 2 buoys, I noticed that 2 other swimmers and myself were the only 3 remaining. Not wanting to come in last place, we all kept moving forward. But for me personally I had to put a little stink on it! Replaying my coaches voice over and over again in my mind,

Stroke, rotate, reach, catch, grab, and breatheeee...

I repeated this to myself as I pushed forward, and with each stroke, I moved closer and closer to the shoreline. As I passed by lifeguards in the safety canoes, I could hear them yelling as if they sensed my resolve,

"Keep moving! You're looking good!"

As I rounded the third buoy, I knew that I was in the home stretch. I was feeling surprisingly good, considering the amount of sleep I had, and my diabetic body was performing very well. As I glanced around the lake, I noticed a swimmer climbing into the safety canoe. No idea what happened to the other person, but I hoped they made it in.

As I passed the final buoy, I knew I had succeeded, a 1.2-mile swim under my belt, and it felt really, really good!

As I exited the water, my polar heart rate monitor read 32 minutes and 140bpm. I was thrilled with my time even knowing that 32 minutes was far too fast of a time for me, but I didn't care. I was out of the water, and that was a victory for me! As I arrived to the bike transition area, I saw my fellow triathlete with the fractured elbow. He asked me if I could strap his helmet, because he couldn't lift his arm. No problem! I imagined the swim aggravated his injury, but in the spirit of competition, he was pushing forward, and so was I.

After transitioning from wetsuit to cycling gear, I was off for the 56-mile bike. Immediately, the route took you up this massive hill. As I pedaled on, I passed many people who had chosen to walk their bikes up the hill. I continued pushing forward, motivated by my spinning instructor's voice yelling,

"Drive that pedal into the ground."

As I reached the top of the hill, I was completely exhausted and out of breath. My heart rate monitor read 170 bpm, a good indication of how challenging the hill was. As I caught my breath and settled into my groove, I remembered the e-mail Dino had sent out the day prior, wishing all the Triathletes good luck, and encouraging us to eat constantly and consume lots of fluids. Excellent advice!

The first 25 miles of the 56-mile bike ride felt good, but throughout the last 36 miles, the humidity had kicked in and the temperature increased to 89 very hot degrees. I stayed faithful to my game plan and resisted the temptation of trying to be a superior.

My made up for this moment definition of (superior) - The temptation of trying to out-do someone that you perceive yourself to be, Better than, More fit than, Stronger than, Younger than. Etc…

You learn early on that a triathlon is a sport where the biggest mistake you can make is trying to judge a participant by their cover. It's never about what appears on the exterior, it's the interior that matters because that is where the heart and real courage lies.

Accepting my God-given abilities, I continued pushing through the remaining 36 miles while consuming water, Gatorade, Fig Newton bars and 3 electrolyte tablets to maintain strength and stability. As I passed through numerous intersections, I received several thumbs up from motorists, and I even received some horn action. I truly appreciated the fan support, and how the sheriff's department patrolled traffic while keeping all participants safe.

During the last 10 miles, I pushed myself very hard while averaging 18 miles per hour. As I approached the finish line, I could hear my girlfriend yelling my name, well not quite!

"Good job Bob," she jokingly yelled.

I knew that she was happy, and I was ecstatic with my time of 3 hours 24 minutes.

My thoughts were if I could maintain this same speed in the full Ironman, I would finish the 112-mile bike around 7 hours. Yet another goal I had set for myself.

After transitioning from my bike to run gear, I checked my blood sugar level before heading out to complete the 13.1-mile run. My glucose read 110, and the build-up of sodium on my skin burned like crazy when I poked my finger.

Silently I wished the pharmaceutical and diabetic supply companies could come up with another way of testing your blood sugars without stabbing your finger.

With the temperature around 87 degrees and the humidity high, most triathletes eat to avoid hitting the wall. I, on the other hand, had packed an adequate supply of Fig Newton bars and GU packets, not only to avoid serious fatigue, but also to avoid getting myself in severe trouble with a hypoglycemic reaction.

As I set out on the run, there it was again, even more intimidating than it appeared less than 3-1/2 hours ago. The same hill that raised my heart rate to 170 as I drove my peddles into the ground. Although running is my strength, the elevation of this hill would challenge even elite runners. Approaching this beast, I knew I would feel every single pound of the pavement. As I began running up the hill, some of the spectators that lined the road shouted out words of encouragement, while many simply shook their heads and stared at each runner as if we were crazy. As I reached the top of the hill, I thought of doing a Rocky celebration, but with an elevated heart rate, I had absolutely no energy.

I was now reduced to a simple shuffle of the feet, and I realized I had attacked the hill excessively hard and a price to pay for showboating awaited me. After mentally focusing on my breathing, I slowed my heart rate down and resumed running at my 9-minute per mile pace.

Once I found my rhythm, I began passing many people I had seen exiting the transition area some 5 minutes earlier than I. But looking at their body language as I passed by, they were obviously paying a price for something. Was it the hill? Did they go out too hard on the bike or the swim? Maybe it was their training or nutrition. These were some of the thoughts and perceptions that occupied my mind during the first 7 miles.

From mile 8, through mile 10, I struggled to hold my gait. Although I was hydrating and eating constantly, nothing seemed to help. I started to feel lightheaded, and because I believed it was somehow related to my diabetes, I made the decision to walk the entire mile 11, and it proved to be worth it. I resumed running a strong mile 12 and 13 en-route to completing my very first Half Ironman Triathlon in 6 hours 32 minutes. Crossing the finish line and hearing the announcer state, "Aaron Perry from Madison," made me feel like a true champion. My heart rate average was 157, and my post-race glucose was 142.

After a brief celebration with some of the other triathletes, I packed up my gear and headed home. During the 2-1/2-hour ride, my girlfriend called her family and friends to inform them I had completed the event. Everyone extended their congratulations and seemed happy for me. Excited and thrilled with my efforts, I remember stating,

"This training stuff really works!"

But deep down inside, I was feeling funny about the 1.2-mile swim. It seemed too "easy" and even though I was the last swimmer to finish, my time of 32 minutes was far too fast. Upon returning to Madison, I checked the Internet to confirm my swim time and place.

Just as I thought, I came in last place with a time of 32 minutes. I consulted with other veteran triathletes who had also participated in the High Cliff Ironman to gauge their perspective on the swim distance. Not to my surprise, many elite endurance athletes also believed the swim was not an official 1.2 miles, but more like a 0.7-mile swim.

Believing that I had yet to officially swim more than a mile, I allowed insecurity regarding the Ironman swim to dominate my thinking. After speaking with my swim coach about this issue, he assured me that I had swam more than a mile numerous times during class. My coach also informed me that things would get more difficult in less than a week when our swim lessons would move from Lake Wingra to the much larger and deeper Lake Monona, the actual sight for the Ironman Triathlon swim.

With 5 solid days of swimming and a total of 8 miles completed, I had regained my confidence in the water and could not wait for the following Monday to arrive to begin swimming in Lake Monona.

Following a weekend that consisted of a 90-mile bike ride and a 15-mile run, Monday had arrived, and I was feeling very fit and ready to take on Lake Monona for the first time. After changing into my wetsuit, I approached the water and immediately recognized the 2-foot swells, the result of a warm but very windy afternoon.

As Mark gathered all the swimmers, a total of 15 altogether, he gave us his instructions, and into the water we went. Within minutes, I began to struggle with the waves. The group began to slowly pull away and out of sight from where I was located. I attempted to swim through the waves but found my level of experience to be no match for the water. As Mark approached me from the rear in his canoe I heard him say,

"Aaron, are you alright?"

Unable to utter a word because I had swallowed so much water, I recall swimming towards the canoe with the intentions of climbing inside for fear of drowning. As I swam towards the canoe, Mark stated something I will never forget,

"Aaron, I have to look out for the greater good of the group and not one individual. Why don't you swim back to shore?"

I had finally reached the canoe and was attempting to grab hold of it when, without hesitation, Mark paddled away nearly slicing my head open with his paddle. I don't believe Mark realized my intentions were to climb into the canoe. I attempted to yell for him to stop, but the waves smashing into my face resulted in me swallowing a large amount of water. Watching Mark paddle away from me and towards the other swimmers sent me into a panic. There I was, 100 - 150 feet from shore and in 75-foot deep water with rough waves.

Completely exhausted and struggling to breath, I immediately reflected back to something Mark had drilled in my head. He stated,

"Aaron, you will never drown in a wetsuit, and if you panic, just flip over on your back and catch your breath."

I was not only panicking, but for a few short and intense moments, I believed I would actually drown.

Refusing to go out like that, the survivor in me completely took over my being. My courage was on the shoreline, and I was going to finally claim it. I flipped over on my back and within seconds, I slowed my hyperventilating. After calming myself down, I flipped back over to resume swimming, but quickly realized I had drifted another 20 to 30 feet away from shore. The view of the Monona Terrace seemed miles away as I began swimming back. I was relieved when I realized that I was swimming with the direction of the waves and with each stroke, I began moving closer and closer to claiming my courage. I managed to flip over on my back one additional time for a brief rest before finally making it safely to shore. Thrilled, nervous, scared and happy were all the emotions I was experiencing as a result of making it back to shore and being able to actually stand up.

With quivering hands, I struggled taking my wetsuit off. I also remember laughing out loud at what had just occurred. Of all the angry emotions I had felt being abandoned by my coach, the only comment I uttered was to myself,

"Aaron, mother nature kicked your booty today."

Ironically I found humor in this frightening episode of my journey to the Ironman. The psychological impact of this experience, seemed to strengthen my resolve and helped convince me that no matter what happen during the 2.4-mile swim, I would not drown. This was a major turning point in my swim training because I had finally claimed my confidence! I now believed I had the power to withstand anything that I faced. My desire to get back into Lake Monona was suddenly strong, but I needed to learn new techniques to swim in rough water. I called Mark when I returned home, but received no answer. I left a detailed message for him to call me so I could schedule a one-on-one lesson with him in Lake Monona. Mark never returned any of my 5 subsequent phone calls, thus ending our relationship.

With 55 days remaining for the Ironman, I accepted that Mark had taken me as far as he could as a coach, and the rest of my journey would be up to me. After all, I hired him to teach me how to swim, and he did! Now it would be up to me to teach myself how to swim 2.4 miles, and I had less than 2 months to make it happen.

CHAPTER 9

Staring Hatred In The Eyes

I began aggressively swimming in Lake Monona on a daily basis, and with each swim I ventured out further and further into the lake. I continued swimming daily until I began experiencing symptoms of an ear infection. After seeking medical attention through Dean Medical Urgent Care, and while waiting to see a doctor, I noticed a wall calendar. It was at this time that I realized I had been swimming for 27 straight days.

After being diagnosed with an ear infection, I was encouraged to stop swimming for 2 days and complied with the doctor's orders. I returned to the lake following this brief break, ear infection and all, but now armed with some prescribed eardrops and earplugs. I continued swimming during the week, while cycling and running on the weekends.

With 30 days remaining for Ironman, I set out early on a Saturday morning for what would be my last 112-mile ride before Ironman. I had planned to follow up the bike ride with a 10-mile run.

It was a beautiful summer morning, and the temperature was expected to reach around 88 degrees. I had packed plenty of fluids and stashed some money to stop at the local gas station in Mt. Horeb for a lunch break. I had figured around mile 70 would be a good time to take my break. As I left Madison, I didn't see many cyclists on the road. I arrived in Verona 40 minutes later and linked up with several female cyclists from Milwaukee, who were also training for the Ironman. They looked like seasoned triathletes, but during the ride from Verona to Mt. Horeb, they disclosed that this would be their 1st Ironman Triathlon. From the looks of their physiques, and from the power they were displaying, I believed they would have no problem making the bike cutoff. Approximately 30 miles into the ride, as we passed through the town of Cross Plaines, they had increased their distance.

"These ladies were serious about their cycling."

Within minutes they were out of sight, and I was riding solo again. After completing the first loop, I decided to stop in Verona for a quick snack. I had been riding for 3 hours 24 minutes and was on pace to complete the 112-mile ride within 7 hours. After finishing off the peanut butter and jelly sandwich and washing it down with water and Gatorade, I was back in the saddle. Although the sun was cooking my caramel colored skin, I felt pretty good. As I approached Mt. Vernon for the second time, I turned onto Route 92. This is the part of the Ironman route that many triathletes didn't care for very much because it seemed only 5 inches separated us from the motorists. Not much room for error on either part.

As I was peddling forward, hugging the shoulder of the road and trying to hold a 17 mph pace, I could hear this vehicle approaching me from the rear.

"They're taking their sweet and precious time passing," I thought to myself.

Thinking that I'm occupying too much room on the road, I glanced over my shoulder to see why this vehicle wasn't passing me. From first glance I could see that an older male was driving, no big deal.

Another 10 seconds passed but this vehicle hadn't passed me. I glanced over my shoulder a second time because I had a sense that the vehicle was getting too close to me. After making eye contact with the driver, and for no reason whatsoever, he laid on the horn!

Initially startled, my first reaction was nearly veering off the shoulder of the road. As I continued on, my Threat Assessment was very high and I intended to get a license plate number from this person who was now harassing me. Not having much room to negotiate on the road, I motioned with my left hand for this individual to pass. He instead pulled alongside of me and began to yell,

"Get off my road!"

The fact that his passenger side window was the only one lowered and the tone of his voice was a strong indication that he was seeking a confrontation. While yelling at me, he also turned the front end of his vehicle toward my bike. I attempted to ignore this idiot while trying to stay focused on keeping my bike from rolling off the shoulder of the road and down the embankment.

As I continued peddling, I saw a driveway leading up to a farmhouse and intended to seek refuge there, but this jerk once again pulled along side of me still ranting and raving out loud. It seemed that as I made repeated attempts to ignore this person, he must have felt empowered by his assumption that I feared him. As he pulled slightly ahead of me his vehicle came to a complete stop. Unsure of his intentions I stopped peddling my bike, and unclipped my shoes in preparation to defend myself.

Staring evil in its eyes, I finally drew a line in the sand. I dismounted my bike, looked at this jerk and I stated very loudly,

"Leave me alone!

He looked at me with this irritated, screwed up look of confusion and drove away.

During this entire encounter, I had noticed many vehicles passing from the opposite direction, but either they didn't realize what was going on, or they didn't care. Maybe it was business as usual in rural Wisconsin. But it didn't matter anymore because my spirit had been wounded. While peddling like crazy to complete the last 40 miles, I began to cringe as vehicles approached from the rear and was constantly looking over my shoulder. I was very disturbed and didn't understand what motivated this confrontation. After linking up with 3 other cyclist who were from the Chicago area, my paranoia subsided a bit as we rode back to Madison in a pack. One of the gentlemen from Chicago asked me how it was going and my only response was,

"I've had better days."

During the ride back to Madison, they talked about how much they loved the route, while I on the other hand wanted so badly to contradict what they were saying about this route, but I kept my feelings to myself.

As I listened to how they praised the beauty of rural Wisconsin, I wondered how it was that we traveled along the same path but had completely different experiences and views. How could our desire to become an Ironman be so equal, but our journeys have nothing in common. How could they finish the bike ride with happiness in their hearts yet I had anger in mine?

What message or fundamental lesson was God attempting to help me gain?

Arriving back in Madison, I wanted to vent to my best friend and soul mate about the anger I had inside, but I instead said a prayer and asked God for clarity.

Reflecting back, I realized I had begun to compare these negative experiences on the Ironman bike route to several past traumatic experiences of my life. Heartbroken but determined to succeed was a feeling I recalled harboring when my mother passed away. Now this! There I was once again saddened with the fact that my spirit had been wounded, and my journey and desire to become an Ironman had been knocked off center.

After praying to God for strength, he directed me to my late mother's message, and once again, I found strength. My mother stated,

"Son, don't try to fix this, let it be rough for awhile and one day you will understand and mature from it".

What my mother wanted me to gain from these experiences was to simply understand that sometimes in life, there are no answers. Just pray, just grow, and one day you will just be better!

After taking a 2-day retreat with my girlfriend, she helped me to see all of the good that this life still has in waiting. I emerged from this retreat with a new spirit that humbled and reassured me that during difficult times, all I had to do was put it in God's hands.

CHAPTER 10

The Ability to Finish

With less than 30 days before the Ironman Triathlon, I had a renewed spirit that wouldn't be broken. I decided on a 2-week taper, which left me with 2 weeks of training.

From August 18, 2005, until September 1, 2005, I swam a total of 10-miles in Lake Monona, biked a total 270-miles, and I averaged over 40-miles of running each week. Needless to say, this was the most demanding 2 weeks of training I had put my diabetic body through all year, and it was also some of the most rewarding.

September 1, 2005, had arrived, and I began tapering off. I accepted the fact that there was absolutely nothing more I could do to physically prepare myself for the world's toughest endurance event set to take place in less than 10 days. The city of Madison and the surrounding communities had begun to catch the Ironman fever. Professional athletes had begun arriving in town, and the city of Madison Streets Department began posting street closure notices.

On September 6, 2005, downtown Madison and the Monona Terrace were completely invaded by Ironman North America. But the one addition that had gotten my attention the most was seeing the large orange buoys being placed in Lake Monona. I now had a good idea of what the Ironman swim route would be, and although this day was also my birthday; my celebration was on hold until after the big event.

In the final 72 hours leading up to Ironman, I had participated in numerous workshops hosted by professionals such as Paula Newby Frasier a 12-time Ironman Triathlete. I visited the Ironman Village formerly the Monona Terrace and I tried on some of the latest triathlon gear, and experimented with some of the newest high tech cycling training modules and assimilators on the market.

On September 8, 2005, Gatorade hosted a 2-day Ironman swim; an event in which they stored all the triathlete's personal items while we practiced on the actual swim route with buoys in place. On September 9, 2005, I took part in the Gatorade swim, an experience I had anticipated. Putting on my wetsuit, starting my polar heart monitor watch and jumping into the lake to swim with triathletes from around the world was unbelievable!

As I began swimming, I remembered approaching the first buoy and finally feeling like I belonged. After rounding each buoy thereafter to complete the first loop, I decided to head in. As I exited the water, my time read 54 minutes. This was a proud moment for me as I remembered my yearlong struggle to claim my courage in the water. I was very relieved to finally confirm to myself that I could swim 1.2 miles, and although my time of 54 minutes worried me a little, I knew that completing two loops at 54 minutes a piece would have me out of the water in 1 hour 48 minutes, and I would be fine with that.

On September 9, I spoke with an African-American male and Sports Director with Channel 3 news. I shared with him the possibility that I could make history by being the first insulin-dependent Africa-American to complete the Ironman. He sounded very excited and happy for me and he stated,

"I want this story. The city of Madison needs to hear this story."

He informed me that he and his camera crew would meet me at the Gatorade swim location on the following day, September 10, 2005. Excited at the thought of being interviewed, I called home and shared the information with family and friends.

The following morning, I arrived as we had discussed, but he was a no show. I called him numerous times but received no return call. Disturbed by his lack of professionalism, I proceeded to contact Channel 27 News, a competitor of channel 3, and I was connected to news anchor Christa Dubil. After explaining my story, Mrs. Dubil stated,

"Aaron, I'm going to make you a star."

She arranged to have reporter Shawn Ryan meet me for an interview at 6:00 am outside the Ironman Village/ Monona Terrace. Mrs. Dubil spoke to me from the heart, and she expressed real feelings towards my goal. Therefore, I knew Channel 27 would follow through.

As I proceeded to the bike check-in area, I was overwhelmed at the sight of 2,100 bikes. If anyone had ever questioned whether or not the Ironman event was considered a big time sporting venture, all they needed to do was visit the Ironman Village.

After attending the Ironman traditional pasta supper, it was time to head home for a final check of my inventory. Arriving home, I was very methodical about making sure I didn't forget anything, but I still had that "Did I forget something?" feeling that drives athletes' nuts. Upon completing my equipment checklist, I looked at the clock and the time was 8:00 pm. While talking to my girlfriend I stated,

"Honey, I'm very nervous about tomorrow."

She looked at me and softly stated,

"You can do this Aaron; I know you can, because I believe in you."

With less than 12 hours before the official start of the Ironman Wisconsin Triathlon, my confidence was in need of a boost, but deep down inside I accepted that I had put myself in a position to succeed by making many lifestyles changes and overcoming many obstacles. After thinking about all the accomplishments I had achieved over the course of one year, I stated to my girlfriend,

"You're right honey, I can do this."

Prior to turning in for what would certainly be a long night, I said a prayer to God, and following my prayer; this is the conversation I had with my body and soul,

"Tomorrow I will ask something of you that I have never asked before. I'm asking for you to give me everything you have to get me to the finish line, and I promise that at any point throughout the race, if you feel that we cannot go forward, I will stop."

At 4:30 a.m. the alarm awakes me, and September 11, 2005, had finally arrived. I checked my blood sugars level, which registered 135. I gave myself an injection of 5-units of Humalog Insulin, then showered and ate a small breakfast consisting of 2 bagels with peanut butter and a glass of orange juice. After gathering my special needs bags I was headed to the Ironman Village/Monona Terrace. My girlfriend and her family had planned to meet up with me prior to the swim start.

Upon arriving in downtown Madison, I immediately noticed how lights from the Wisconsin State Capital illuminated the entire area along Martin Luther King Jr. Boulevard. A perfect backdrop for what I had hoped would be a perfect day. As I walked my special needs bag to the designated area outside of the State Capitol, I followed the steady stream of Ironman veterans, age groupers and family members back towards the Ironman Village. I saw my girlfriend's beautiful face right away. She was standing atop the Monona Terrace with her family, and I thanked them for coming to support me. I showed my girlfriend the beautiful card she had given me for motivation, and I informed her of my intentions to carry it with me all day. I think she may have shed a tear.

It was 6:00 a.m. when I saw the Channel 27 news television van pull along side the City County building. A young man exited the van and introduced himself as Mr. Shawn Ryan. Following a brief introduction, we discussed the Ironman Triathlon while walking down to the Lake.

Shawn interviewed me while I changed into my wetsuit, and I began to feel like a celebrity as many of the thousand spectators watched my interview.

I even saw a few kids standing with a pencil and paper in hand, but they never asked for an autograph.

"Smart kids! They knew I was an amateur and not one of the pros."

Shawn asked questions about my quest to make history as the first African-American insulin-dependent diabetic worldwide to complete the Ironman Triathlon, and I shared with him how much of an honor this would be. He advised me that he would be present at different locations throughout the day shooting footage of me. I thanked Channel 27 news for this opportunity to share my story, and I proceeded to the starting area for the 2.4-mile swim.

Although I was a participant in the event, I was amazed at how many people lined the swim area and the upper deck of the Monona Terrace. It was truly something special to witness, and I was in it.

With minutes remaining before the canon sounded, all 2,146 swimmers from all around the world had worked their way into the lake. While looking around in amazement, I saw former New York Jets player Al Toon, who was the master of ceremony. As I proceeded to give him the thumbs up,

"Boom"

The canon went off and the 2005 Ford Ironman Wisconsin Triathlon was underway. My strategy was to swim to the outside at the beginning and then angle in toward the buoys. I stayed focused on my plan and didn't exert myself during the first loop. My toes had begun cramping about 30 minutes into the swim, so I stopped kicking my legs and stroked hard with my arms. I resumed kicking after the cramping subsided and felt surprisingly good after completing the first loop. I proceeded to stroke my arms and kick my legs a little harder on the second loop because I began to believe that I was going to make it in. As I rounded the last and final loop, I knew I would make it. With each stroke, I moved closer and closer to earning the right to advance to the 112-mile bike. As I approached the shoreline, I could hear the music and the loud cheering from the crowd.

Finally, there I was, getting out of the water and pumping my fist as if I had won something. With a time of (1 hour 55 minutes 30 seconds), I was overjoyed at what I had accomplished. Waiting at the top of the shoreline was Reporter Shawn Ryan. He could see the joy in my face, and he asked how my blood sugars were and I happily replied,

"My blood sugars feel a little low, so when I get to the transition room, I plan to eat a few fig Newton bars."

Running up the helix and seeing and hearing all the spectators cheering was a feeling that I wish everyone could experience in their lifetime. Arriving to the T-1 swim-to-bike transition, I was on cloud nine. After changing into my cycling gear, I was running out of the transition area to get my bike. Although I could hear many people yelling my name, I tried to stay focused. After mounting my bike, I headed down the helix and onto John Nolen Drive to begin the 112-mile ride that included 6,900 feet of total hill climbing.

Traveling down John Nolen drive was a familiar sight as I had trained on the route throughout the past 5 months, a bit of an advantage, but I was fine with that. I arrived in Verona in 50 minutes. Happy with my time, I pushed on to begin the loop. As I traveled through areas of Mt. Vernon and Mt. Horeb, I briefly thought of the negative experiences I had encountered, but I was on a mission and nothing was going to alter my destiny. As I completed the first loop, I saw my girlfriend standing near the corner waving at me. She had managed to make her way out to Verona just to see me, and I appreciated it, and I appreciated her!

I stopped for a lunch break at mile 60, but concerned with my time, I made it very brief. I quickly completed my 3rd glucose check of the day, which read 180! As I began the second loop, I began experiencing some cramping. I took several salt tablets and consumed more fluids. Within minutes, the cramping had subsided, and I was now passing through Cross Plains. I was within minutes of the Old Sauk Pass and Timberline Road, the highest degree of difficulty of all the hills. Climbing the hills on the first loop at mile 38 was challenging, but I was now approaching the hills for the second time at mile 76 and with fatigued legs, I knew it was going to hurt.

Approaching Old Sauk Pass Road, which had a fairly steep incline, I stayed in the saddle the entire climb because that had worked during my training rides as well as on the first loop. As I made it to the top of the hill, I was now focused on the approaching Timberline Road, which according to many Triathletes boasts one of the highest degrees of difficulty of all Ironman events. I questioned what strength I had left for the Midtown and Whalen roads, but I pressed forward. I had consumed a GU pack for any energy I could find, and I had hoped it would kick in as I approached the base of Timberline Road. But with little energy, I began driving my pedals into the ground, and I crept closer and closer until I reached the top. Knowing that I would not have to see Timberline road for another year, I wanted to celebrate, but I had Midtown and Whalen roads remaining. As I approached the Midtown hill, I stayed with my strategy of remaining in the saddle and as I begun climbing the most difficult hill of all. I simply dropped my head and pushed as hard as I could. I remember this spectator shouting,

"You are killing my hill, way to go man!"

I fed off of his energy and in many ways I truly needed to hear that kind of positive support from a rural Wisconsin resident. This stranger's comment set the tone for the remainder of my bike ride. As I passed through Verona, I had apparently missed my cheering section. My girlfriend said that I must have been very focused, because they screamed very loud and I didn't even notice. With 17-miles remaining, I began to experience severe cramps in my legs and chest. Completely out of glycogen, I turned this over to God, and he came through for me. After saying a prayer, I was given a boost of glycogen that sustained me over the remainder of my ride.

As I neared the Monona Terrace, I knew that I had made the bike cutoff time. Riding up the helix to complete the 112-mile ride, I was happy to be getting off the bike.

(7 hours 54 minutes 45 seconds) and I was ok with that. (Next up T-2).

Transitioning from my bike to run gear, I knew that all I had to do was average 13-minute miles for 26.2 more miles, and I would become an Ironman. As I exited the transition area, I was happy to see my love, my life. She asked how I felt,

"Surprisingly good I replied."

I gave her a kiss and told her I would see her in 5 to 6 hours. As I began to run, I felt as if I had gotten stronger. I had now been participating for over 10-hours straight and wanted to push it a little, but I feared a physical meltdown. I managed to stay within my game plan and as the hours passed and nighttime appeared, I began to pay close attention to my watch.

After completing the first loop of 13.1-miles, I headed back out for the last and final loop.

My time was a (3 hour 34 minute) split. My 5th glucose check of the day registered 165!

Constantly keeping a close eye on the time, I began to feel it. Thirteen more miles I stated while continuing to whisper to myself,

"Keep moving forward."

As I passed the lake path, I looked over to see Frank, the 78-year-old Ironman Triathlete going in the opposite direction. I looked at my watch and imagined he knew he would not make it in by the midnight cut off time. But being a veteran Ironman, I knew he would not give up, and neither would the spectators leave until he crossed the finish line. It was now approximately 11:10 pm, and as I turned the corner from the Civic Center, I could hear the roar of the crowd from a distance. Two more miles I said out loud as I pushed on. As I approached

Carroll Street, my eyes had begun to tear up. With each step I took the crowd got louder and louder. I fought to hold in my emotions because approximately 364 days earlier when I had began my journey, I had poor control of my diabetes, I didn't know how to swim, I weighed 220 lbs with 28% body fat, I had never ridden my bike more than 20 miles, and I had never run more than 6 miles. And as I approached the final 100 yards, I thought about all the accomplishments I had achieved over the course of one year, and suddenly, there I was, slapping high fives with the spectators while looking around for my girlfriend. I wanted to pull her over the barricade and have her cross the finish line with me, but with 10,000 spectators screaming, I knew she could see me from wherever she was. As I approached the finish line, I pumped my fist in the air and screamed,

"Yes, I did it!"

On September 11, 2005, at 11:35 pm with a time of (16 hours 34 minutes and 57 seconds), I became histories first African-American insulin-dependent diabetic to complete the Ironman Triathlon. With God's blessing, I amazed myself...

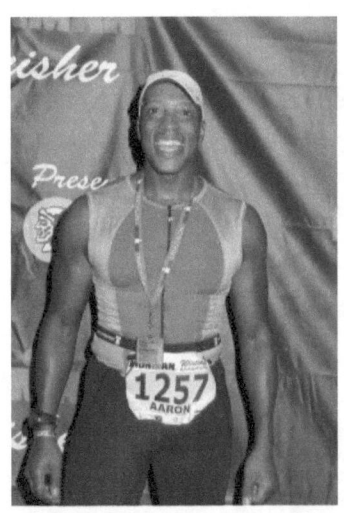

Aaron G. Perry

Ironman Triathlete

Being a former police officer, September 11th already held a special place in my heart. And now this day has become a day of personal achievement, that's filled with pride and great satisfaction that I will carry with me forever.

To all who inspired, coached, mentored, encouraged, and yes, even angered me into achieving this momentous goal, please know that the medal that was placed around my neck in some way or another was put there because of what you said or did to push me where I needed to go. And because of that, I thank you.

www.ingramcontent.com/pod-product-compliance
Lightning Source LLC
Chambersburg PA
CBHW021253280526
45784CB00005B/2352